Alzheimers
Willie's Story

Alzheimers
Willie's Story

Cathy Long Hester

To order additional copies of this book, contact:
Xlibris Corporation
1-888-795-4274
www.Xlibris.com
Orders@Xlibris.com
103549

INTRODUCTION

This is a diary that I have wanted to write about my mom for a long time. She has Alzheimer's, but she has had it for a long time. We as a family did not know. The signs and symptoms were there, but we just thought nothing of it. My father was not an easy man to live with when they were first married. But as the years went on, I wondered if my father knew she was sick and kept it from us until she got so bad we got to notice it ourselves.

I really wish I had noticed her condition before she got so bad, but I married and moved away. Daddy kept her condition hidden; he made out the grocery list. Even though my sister took her to the grocery store, Mother would go by the list that Daddy had written out and would not get anything that was not on the list. Now she would get some things Daddy would not mind so much. But as time went on, Mother would not even go to the store anymore; her behavior would not let her.

One thing I was proud of was that she wrote a book about her life growing in Columbia, Arkansas. That will be good reading as soon as I can put the events in order.

My mother was a peacemaker.

My father died on June 6, 2004. He had several health problems, but I think he willed himself to live as long as he did. My father was a hard man to please, for me anyway.

But he covered my mom's condition. So after Daddy died, my mom was very stubborn. She didn't like anything and wanted things her way.

So here goes

My brother Doug stayed with Mother during the week. I drove up on weekends and stayed. During the course of Mother's disease, Doug had heart surgery and my sister and I had shoulder surgery.

We got Mother a new trailer—well, not a brand-new one, but new to Mom. It was so much bigger and had two bathrooms.

Saturday, 09/16/06. That is the weekend I came up to take care of my mom. It was the usual routine: she eats raisin bran, a piece of bread, a fourth of an apple, and vanilla wafer, six of them, with ice cream in the middle with cool whip on top three times a day. Now that sounds so gross, but she still eats, so we just let her eat it. We know that one of these days she will stop eating. Also could be bed bound, so we are so thankful that she is ambulatory.

I stay Saturday and the night also. Well Sunday morning, when I went into her bedroom, she was on the floor. I don't know for how long. I got her up off the floor, but it took me a long time; she could not help me. Then her balance was so off she almost fell several times. My sister, who relieves me, came, and she noticed how she was not acting right also. Mom was leaning to the right when she walked with her walker, you had to be walking on her right to support her. My sister and brother took her to see the nurse-practitioner who works for her regular MD. She ordered an ultrasound of her abdomen. After the blood work was so off her liver function. So the ultrasound showed that she had lesions in her liver and her right kidney. My mother has a chronic urinary infection problem. This is a problem in her family. My aunt was on dialysis, and my uncle had colon cancer and stroke. Oh, and also abdominal cancer. So our family history is sort of grim. Mother now is so imputation. She wants to know what time it is.

Saturday, 09/30/06. I went to Mother's house; she looked good. She seemed glad to see me; I was so happy. Mom asked me about my girls. Have I heard from them lately? I told her that Jackie was in town and is coming out to see her today. She was so excited. She raised Jackie until she started going to school. Really, she raised Heather also. We had to get her a new couch because I had to start sleeping in the living room. I was afraid to sleep in the bedroom; in case she fell again, I would hear her. Well, she does not like the new couch; she wants the old one put back in the living room. We put the old couch in the bedroom. I told Mom how good the new couch looks. She would just look at me. I told her that when Heather comes down for Thanksgiving she will fall in love with it; again this blank look. Sometimes I look at her and wonder who this woman she may look like my mom is. But she does not act like my mother. I know that this is so hard on our family and other families who have a loved someone with this disease. This disease is so cruel, does not care what race or gender.

Mother loves Josh Turner, the country singer. We bought her the video of "Long Black Train"; she plays it over and over again at first. But now the country music she had to listen to seemed like 24-7 now not so much. I mean drove us crazy with it to the point that I listen to it in the mornings while getting ready for work; well, I watch the videos. Mother wants the video, of course, of Josh Turner's "Your Man." No VHS of that, only DVDs. You know it's so hard to see her that way. She always remembers the bad things that have happened to me. My first husband was abusive to me. Every time I come to stay with her, she brings him up and how he beat me. She will say, "Your dad said not to bring up the bad things that happened in the past." But then she'll bring it up.

10/13/06. I drove up on Friday after work. Mom seemed feebler, and her right hand shook more to me; also, she looked like she lost some weight. I think it confused her, me coming up early. She went to bed and came back out of her room, and I reminded her to take her meds. She went back to bed; she only got up one time. But when my brother got up and left his house, he slammed his truck door, and of course, Mother thought it was time to get up. I told her it was too early to get up. She went back to bed and got up at 8:00 a.m. She told me she didn't want to go back to bed. I told her she didn't have to. I guess she thought I was going to make her go back to bed. That made me feel so bad. I do not want my mother to think I'm mean. So as usual what time it is started at 11:00 a.m. because *The Road Show, The Lawrence Welk Show,* and *Keeping Up.* That really got on my nerves, and then I feel bad. So this goes on until the shows come on. *Yeah!* So then Mother goes to bed. She slept well, only got up once to go to the bathroom.

Sunday morning, 10/15/06. The cat kept me up most of the night as usual. My sister came over to relieve me early, for which I really was glad. Mother was still asleep. I made my sister check on her; she was okay. She finally got up and went to the fridge and started to drink her poop meds, prune juice. I got the juice and only poured two ounces for her to drink. At first I think she was very mad at me, but she got over it quick. I left her in good hands with my sister.

Monday, 10/16/06. My sister called me at work and told me that my mother was collecting urine specimen and had them all lined up in a row. My brother was freaking out, so my sister said she just wanted me to know what was going on!

Saturday, 10/28/06. I got to Mother's at 8:00 a.m. She was eating breakfast. My brother was there. So he was ready to leave; but of course, he was glad to get his money, twenty-five dollars, to stay on the Saturday that I can't come up. Now I always thought that was greedy, but that is my opinion. Mother started in on the time change fall back an hour in the fall of the year. Well if I heard that once, I heard that a hundred times. I was about to pull my hair out plus what time is it. I cleaned so much Saturday ceiling fan, light fixtures, mopped two times, washed curtains. When my oldest brother lived with my mom, he would sneak and smoke in her house, so her house smells, especially in the spare bedroom and bathroom. When I come home, I have to wash my clothes, and the cat has fleas, which we are trying to get rid of, but my other brother has seven or eight dogs that he uses for hunting deer, so the fleas are terrible. Mother brought up the past, as usual, but I told her to please not talk about it, and for once she didn't. She gets so confused about her shows—the times they come on and the channels they come on—that we go over this about twenty times before they come on. I'm so mentally drained; it's all I can do to keep up with it myself after a while. When I changed the clocks back an hour, she did not believe that I changed the clock in her bedroom, so we had to go. And she saw for herself that I had changed the time. Well when her shows were over, she got ready for bed, and she took her meds. But she had to come back in the living room to make sure she had taken her meds. This seems like this happens every time I'm up to take care of her. She wants to eat at 8:00, 12:00 and 4:30, or she wants to put her evening food out to eat at 8:00 p.m. I really have to talk her out of that, and that takes a lot of talking. She is very hardheaded. It's either the disease or the meds she is on for her disease.

Sunday, 10/29/06. Of course, I didn't sleep well. The cat was yowling most of the night, wanting to lie on me, and Mother got up to go to the bathroom only once though. The time change made us both get up early. I was so glad to see my sister this morning. So I left and went over to my daughter's grandmother's house and drank a cup of coffee and ate a cinnamon roll. We talked for a while, then I left coming back home, which is a three-hour drive. Now if people really wanted, they could have me committed. I love to listen to music and drive doesn't mind what kind. I just jam and sing and dance while I drive; I have to do something to keep from going to sleep. Sometimes I get a lead foot, and I try to slow down, but I want to get home! I do my best thinking also when I'm driving home and crying.

When I was in junior and senior high school, I played basketball. Our games were after school, so Mom would have my supper cooked and my overnight bag packed with my uniform and shoes. I found out later that she would cut out my write-ups in the paper telling how many points I scored when I played forward. Then I switched to guard; she would cut out how many rebounds I got. I get very tired driving up, but I need to do this for Mom and Daddy seems like when he died, the family fell apart. All the meanness came out of my brothers. I know Daddy would be so upset. But I think he knew about how the other brother really is.

Saturday, 11/04/06. My sister woke me up with a phone call about 8:00 a.m. Said Mother was very confused this morning. I did not go up to Hot Springs this weekend. Sister said Mother wanted to know when I'm coming over. Mother was trying to call Ms. Schneller on the TV's remote control. I guess she thought I was over at her house. Sister said that my brother said Mother woke up 4:00 a.m. and went in the dark, into the closed bedroom. He asked her, "What are you doing, Mother?" She said she was trying to find a place to sit down. Sister said Mother wanted to talk to me. I got on the phone, and Mother kept telling me about *The Road Show, Keeping Up,* and *The Lawrence Welk Show* is going to be on may not be on next week. I told Mother that if it isn't, we can watch something else. It seems she is so used to me and her watching those shows with her. I guess she is so confused and wants me up there with her. After all, I watch the shows with her. It finally got through to her that I wasn't coming up. It is not good that Mother is getting up and wandering around the house. I will call Mother later on today. Mother is going down today. I called my sister this afternoon; she said that Mother has calmed down some but asks her what time it is and talks about her shows that will be coming on tonight. I told her that we are going to be into a lot of grief before it's over with.

11/13/06. This is my weekend I took over for my sister. I think this was her first time to ever spend the night with Mom. She was exhausted, said the cat kept her up with the mournful crying she does. I told her that was normal for that cat. So she leaves, and it's just Mom and me going pretty good for a while. I cleaned all day; the house was a mess, especially the back bedroom and the bathroom. Well it started what time is it the usual, but she is going down so fast it seems. Mom doesn't remember names of her children or grandchildren. I'm sick this weekend, and it is hard for me to talk. My voice is very hoarse; I just don't feel well. Mother went on about me cutting her toenails. I told her I would after a while. Well, she kept on until I cut those suckers, which is no easy task. She jerks her foot away, saying I hurt her in which I know I did not hurt her.

Later on that evening, Mom got up from the chair and started running toward the bathroom. I said, "Mom, don't forget your walker," She said, "I don't have time," and sure enough, she had a bowel movement all over the floor in the bathroom and all over her clothes. I never saw so much crap in my life. So I cleaned her up, changed her clothes, and had to wash her house shoes. This has not been very good so far; hopefully, in the morning it will be different.

11/14/06. Well, first thing this morning, Mom went for the prune juice. I told her, "Hell no, old woman, do you remember the crap all over the bathroom?" Mom said, "Oh yeah, I did that, didn't I?" So when my sister came to relieve me, I told her to watch her about the prune juice. I had called my sisters the night before and told them what had happened. I kissed Mom good-bye and went back to Crossett.

11/22/06. I have come to spend the Thanksgiving holidays with Mother and to give my other siblings a rest. When I got to my mother's, my brother was at Mom's. All she would talk about was her birthday cake white cake and white icing. She kept reminding me, "I do not like chocolate." Now she said this over and over again. She called my sister and said, "Are you coming over tomorrow? And I want a peach cobbler." Maybe Mom was confused more with me coming up early. I really don't know. My sister came and brought Mom her groceries. Mother ask her if she was coming down Thursday to give her her bath and wash her clothes. I told Mother I could do that, but Mother said she did not think I knew how to wash her clothes and roll her hair. Mother had forgotten that when I would come up on Saturdays before I hurt my arm, I would give her bath and wash her clothes and make her bed. So now I think she thinks I'm not capable to do that.

It will be a fun Thanksgiving. My oldest daughter is coming to spend a few days with us. Heather hasn't seen Mother in a while. This should be fun!

Mother wants a party for her birthday on Friday. So I'll be writing about that soon. So until tomorrow, will be signing off tonight!

11/23/06. Mother got up two times during the night to go to the bathroom. Now I mean when Mother gets, up you know about it; the light comes on and she makes her presence known. So I've been up since 2:00 a.m. Mother slept late, almost nine o'clock. Mother would not let me give her a bath; my sister had to come and give it to her. Mother said I didn't know how. She almost didn't let me wash her sheets and make her bed. Then she goes in to see if I did it right. Heather is here; she can see a big difference in Mom. Mom has really going fast what mind she has, bless her heart. I was sitting on the couch, and Mother looked at me and asked me who I was. I told her who I was, and she said, "Oh!"

Mother would not eat any Thanksgiving regular food, only a piece of bread, raisin bran cereal, and her vanilla wafers and ice cream. She ate this in all three meals. I wish she could remember something of my childhood. My mother does not remember eating regular food; she says, "I don't like that whatever food you mention" even though you know she ate the foods she said she doesn't like. Mother went to bed as usual, but I kept hearing a bumping sound on the wall. I went into Mother's bedroom; she had fallen in a big box and could not get up, so I helped her up. She went to the bathroom, then back to bed.

I was real nervous all night, afraid she would fall.

Now I know everyone will think I'm crazy. Last night—well, early in the morning—I woke up and I could see someone in the kitchen. Now I sleep on the couch. I told Mother to go back to bed and asked her what she was doing up; no answer. I said again, "Mother, go back to bed." Nothing. I got up, went into the kitchen; no one was there. My daughter had gone shopping. She had left at 4:00 a.m. The only thing that I could think it could be was my dad.

I know that sounds stupid, but what else could it be? Some weird things happen in this house. But it doesn't scare me.

11/24/06. This my mother's birthday today. I guess she is excited; hard to tell.

My brother came by and brought her a card. She really wasn't that excited. We will have cake later on. I have noticed that she's drooling more. I guess that goes along with the disease. Will continue later. I know my patience is getting thinner. That makes me feel like a jerk. I know she can't help it, but it is so hard. I pray so much that God will forgive me when I get upset with my mom.

Well, as usual, my mother did not like the mattress cover for her bed that I got her for her birthday. Mother said, "I have one and it works fine," even though the one on her bed is so stretched out and it does not fit her bed anymore. Well we had a talk about it, and I told her that when the bed is made again, the new mattress cover would be on the bed. She didn't like that at all. She kept repeating over and over, "Is Jackie coming into the airport in Little Rock?" Heather kept saying, "No, Grandma, in Fayetteville, and I have to leave Saturday to pick her up." Now this went on at least every five minutes. This is so hard on us all, and it gets on our nerves so bad. Heather said that she is so much worse than the last time she was here last. Mother ate a small piece of her birthday cake. I guess she liked it; she didn't say. I really think she was happy about her birthday.

11/25/06. The day started like every other day. Breakfast only a fourth of the apple she tells me that three times a day not nicely either. Heather left and went to town. Mother didn't think she was coming back. She told me that at least twenty times before Heather got back.

My great-nephew came down with his dog. Mother told me to take the dog and my great-nephew in my car and take them home. I think Mother does not like children anymore. She used to, but the disease has taken that away from her.

Earlier, when my sister came down with my great-nephew, we were talking, and the Jehovah's Witness girl came by. Mother likes her. When my dad was alive, they came at least every other week. My dad was so nice to them and gave them contributions.

Heather left and went back to Fayetteville. I really hated to see her go. One thing I would be here with Mother she has gotten so hateful and aggressive. She will tell me, "Get me this or do this," and not in a nice voice. My mother was so nice in the past, never mean.

Mother wanted to eat at two thirty for her supper. Finally, I let her eat at four o'clock. Then we had a really long and hard talk about her meds. She wanted to take them before six. Well, she took her meds, and she got ready for bed. She went to the bathroom, and I heard this noise, and I knew what it was: she had a bowel movement all over the commode. I cleaned the commode and the floor and the shower curtain. She has to drink her prune juice every morning. She said she was going to bed, then she had to go to the bathroom again. I could tell it was diarrhea especially when I flushed. I told Mother, "No prune juice in the morning." She argued with me that that was not a loose bowel movement. I told her anyway your poop is b.m.

So she is supposed to be going to bed. I took the remote control and was finding what was on TV. Mother comes in, takes the control, and starts looking at the TV. So I start cleaning the house, then she goes to bed. Now I really do not know if she does this on purpose, but I'm beginning to wonder!

12/09/06. I came up early this morning. Mother seems very quiet today; usually she's talking about things I don't want to hear. Her tremors in her right hand are worse. She still can tell you how to fix her apple only a fourth and peel the skin off.

I brought some big Band-Aids for her shin. Mother had a biopsy Thursday and had some moles on her back taken off that did not look good. We will have the results in one week. I still can't get over how quiet Mother is. Tomorrow is another day. I just pray she has a good night of rest.

12/21/06. I drove up from Crossett today. Mother had a MD appointment with the dermatologist. He had to have abridgment of the areas on her right shin area and her back, where the MD took off skin cancer two weeks ago. The area on her leg looked really bad to me. Mother has no tolerance for pain with her disease now. So I had to suggest to the MD to give her more meds to numb her leg, which he did. We are to change her dressing one time a day, wash the areas with soap and water, put antibiotic ointment on the areas, and cover them with Band-Aids. I just hope the boys will do this daily. Mother seems so frail and childlike in the MD's office. It breaks my heart. I will be with her Saturday and Saturday night.

I will write on Saturday about Mother, but if something comes up sooner, I will write.

12/23/06. Got to Mother's house. She was in a good mood, but as the day went on, things got worse. She kept saying she had no money. I explained to her that her money was kept in the bank. She would just look at me with this blank stare on her face. It was so sad. My mother never was concerned about money. But then Daddy always took care of the money. Jackie came over to the house. Mother asked her the first thing, "Do you have any money for me?" Poor Jackie; she just brought me my lunch and visited her grandmother. Jackie was so upset when she left. I told Mother again that her money was in the bank. And then the stare again. I did my usual cleaning and washing of clothes. I think that's how I cope with the way my mother is now. About 2:00 p.m. it started, the times her shows would come on. So that's what we did all afternoon, ask and answer.

When she was eating supper, she got mad at me. When I was getting her bread out of the bread container, I noticed the container was dirty and I started cleaning it. Well, Mother informed me it was not dirty, and I told her yes, it was and I was cleaning it. Well, a look of hatred came over my mother's face like I have never seen before.

Her shows came on, and she was so happy. I really don't like them, but I watch them.

So at 8:30 p.m., she gets ready for bed. Takes her at least thirty minutes.

So we finally get to get ready for bed, the cat and me.

About 1:30 a.m. Mother gets up to the bathroom in which she makes more noise and turns on the lights. Of course, I wake up; this happens at least two times that night.

12/24/06. Wake up at 7:20 a.m. My sister comes to relieve me. Mother gets up; I fix her breakfast. Then she starts in again about the money, so I put her seven one dollar bills in a Christmas card. She seemed to be a little happy but brought up now who was Heather's daddy. I told Mother that I had kids by everybody. Then I told her not to start that; we have had a good weekend. Again the stare. My sister started cooking, and Mother started in on Josh Turner's "Your Man" video. That was my cue to leave and go home.

At 1:30 p.m. my mother called and wanted the girls to come over and put together her DVD player that my oldest sister had given her for Christmas. Mother did not like the DVDs that my sister had gotten her; she just said to take them all back.

12/25/06. I called to wish Mother a Merry Christmas, and my brother said that Mother had taken all the wires out from behind the TV that had hooked up to the DVD. Poor Doug was reading the directions and was going to put it back together. Mother is so childlike now more than ever. Doug said that on Sunday her sister came to visit her. Mother did not know who she was or her youngest sister. I know it breaks their hearts like it does ours.

01/06/07. Well I hoped and prayed that this would be a good day, but I was wrong. Mother has this thing about money. Then all she could bring up was about me getting beat up. Mother would do this in a sneaky way because she knows how I feel about the situation.

So I would tell her, "Don't talk about that," then she would stop for a while, then here it would go again. That really wears you and your patience down. I tried so hard not to get so upset, but I just can't help it. Then she will go on about her shows that come on, what time, and I would say I don't know, then she would tell me which show and what time. So that makes me think she really wants to just see how far she can push you.

Mother just can't get the money that she gave the girls for Christmas. I finally told her that Daddy always gave the grandchildren Christmas money. I also told her that my other sister was in charge of the money and when her money was where she could not give any more money that would be fine not to worry. Mother gets in this drawer and pulls out checks where the doctor had charged her, and Daddy had written the checks. I looked at the checks, which were dated 1995. I tried to explain to her the date on the checks. Now I should have known better; this disease is so stressful on everyone. Mother gets worse every time I come up. I went out to get my cell phone charger and charged up my phone. Mother tried to open the door. It is dark outside. I said, "Mother, what are you doing?" She answered, "I was seeing what you went outside for." I explained for my cell phone charger. "Well, where is it?" So she came over and had to look at the charger. She kept asking me earlier if she could take her medicine early. I kept telling her no, not until 7:00 p.m. She would say, "I think I'll take my medicine now." I would say, "Not until 7:00 p.m." I was so happy when she could take her pills. Lord, I pray she sleeps well tonight.

01/26/07. I haven't been to Mother's in three weeks. But my sisters tell me Mother is getting so much worse. Seems like she is into changing clothes several times a day. She is falling even more. I was on the way to see her and had a wreck. So it's going to be a while before I can see her. I have to rely on my sisters for my information on her condition. My oldest sister was wondering what stage of the disease she is in. At this time, I really do not know.

There are so many. This disease affects its victims so awfully. Why can't someone find a cure for this disease? The things your loved ones do are heartrending. And you can't do a damn thing about it.

01/27/07. I called my sister, and she said today was a good day for Mother. She fixed her meals today and did not want any help. Said she liked to fix her own meals. She talked about the past a lot. Was a good day.

When I came up for Thanksgiving in November 24, 2007, the girls came down to stay with us. It was so funny; we couldn't get the wire that holds the legs together on the turkey, so we called my niece's boyfriend to come and help. The first thing we said was, "Wash your hands," and he did. He got the wire undone, and we cooked all day. Mother just looked at us like we were crazy. The girls are going shopping the day after. I may go, so I called my oldest brother to come and stay with my mother. I was so happy that we are all together. That night my great-niece came and spent the night with us. She slept with me on the couch. The girls ran to the older trailer and got some stuff. They got scared about something and ran back to the other trailer, where I was. Heather said that Daddy said that he would haunt her because of her pilfering. Well, all of a sudden, the cabinet opened and a bowl flew out, and the light over the stove that was off came on. Well that night the cat started yowling. My great-niece rose from the bed as I also did; she put her arm in front of me and shushed the cat.

The girls got up early at about 4:00 a.m. and went shopping. My brother came over, and we drank coffee and had a great conversation. I'm glad we talked because I lost him in 2010; he coded on the dialysis machine.

We as a family had a good relationship; not at all with two of the family.

Three years of observation on her condition shows how she has progressed in her condition. Got deleted somehow. I'm so upset. All the work I've put into this is gone. Nothing I can do about it now. I cried so much over this.

Mother does not know any of us anymore. She is feeble, falls some. You have to watch her in the bathroom because sometimes she will play with her feces. She gets the sundowner's bad, wants her glasses and her clothes.

I would often get calls from my oldest sister we call sister. She would tell me some things mother had done. I would drive up on several occasions and stay with Mother. I especially stayed during Thanksgiving. We would have a blast. One year she thought we gave her a birthday party. You see, as before, I may have mentioned that before. Mother did eat some of the food. Not much.

I know that in the years 2008 and 2009, before my oldest sister became guardian over Mother, my niece and great-niece would stay at night with Mother. My other sister would pay them, which was okay because Mother can take the last bit of energy from you. You are so mentally and physically drained. I would continue to drive up on the weekends. I would pay my great-niece when I couldn't come. She would also relieve my oldest sister on Saturday that I didn't come also on Sundays, I think.

If the family was at good times with each other, I could write other things, but you get afraid because you never know what they will do. This is a big mess.

05/30/09. Mother was glad to see me. I don't think she knew who I was. That's okay. As long as she knows I love her. She's wondering about Willie. I ask her, "Where and what are you doing?" She says, "Just pilfering." At least she's honest. She wants to go to Mount Pine.

My great-nephew came to visit. Mother just closes her eyes. I guess she thinks he's not there. My great-nephew and I cooked today. We had pasta and salad; we had a great time. We get along so well. Whenever I'm at Mother's, he comes and sees me.

Mother ate a great breakfast. Yvonne said that Mother ate oatmeal and bacon and also a half piece of toast.

Seems like Mother's appetite is not as good to me today. Mother usually can't wait for us to fix her meals, but not so much today.

I talked with my other sister, and she said that when her bath Mother doesn't look like it to her. I said okay, but to me yes. I haven't seen her in three weeks.

The court case is still on the twenty-second of June; I dread that. I don't want to get involved in that.

Mother's shows didn't come on; that was a night of awful.

Mother was up and down. I'm going to bed, then she was getting up. I'm going to watch some TV then. She's going back to bed. This happened about five times. Now she's in bed ten till nine. I will get some sleep, I hope. We shall see. Well, she didn't sleep as well as we thought.

2/19/10. I found that Mother went to bed after my sister left. I got her up because it was time for the news. She got up and watched the news and *Wheel of Fortune*. She seems more bent over. But she still walks. Ate her supper, then went to bed. I had to get her teeth and put them in the container and put it the kitchen. Then I have to get clothes, put them in the other bedroom, then tell Mother I'm washing them.

She got up a couple of times during the night; thank goodness I was tired. Earlier I had gotten Dale's and my plots. There are three plots, and I will be buried in the middle by Mother. She slept pretty well during the night. She always gets up at least two times during the night.

02/20/10. Mother says, "Can I get up now?" I said sure, fixed her breakfast, and my sister came to relieve me.

04/09/10. Got to Mom, and it has started; she is horrible. "Is my clothes done yet?" she asks. We have to hide them, or she will get up during the night dressed. It's after 8:00 p.m., and she's still up. Hope she goes to bed soon and quits asking me "Who are you?" Drives me crazy.

04/10/10. Mother ate her breakfast pretty well; she took her meds. She always asks me, "Who are you talking to?" I'm trying to talk on the phone, and she starts talking louder. Then she says again, "Who are you talking to?" I would tell her she was too nosy.

Mother said she didn't feel well, so I told her to go lie down for a while, maybe she will feel better At 12:00 she ate lunch and did eat pretty well; she loves her bananas. Mom will now be able to watch her Westerns, then she will eat her supper, and the fight to begin taking off her clothes. "No, Momma, we take them off at night." She'll say, "Oh, that's right. I'm so stupid." I would say, "Mother, you are not stupid. Your brain has your memories mixed up sometimes."

05/21/10. Well, I'm at Mom's. She said, "Who are you? Where do you live? Do you have any children?" I lied to Mother and said, "No children." I that I did that, but she doesn't understand. She thinks my daughter Heather is her daughter. Heather is the chosen one. Mother didn't eat her cereal at supper, so I called my sister and told her I wasn't giving Mother the vanilla wafers, ice cream, and cool whip for breakfast. I will feed her the cereal. She'll eat that. This is so terrible; she is more stooped over. It seems that every time I come up she is worse. I ask the Lord to help me. I have no patience anymore. My usual "I don't understand this disease." That's my mom who loved me so much. She slept well; I didn't. I woke up, couldn't think where I was.

05/22/10. She got up and said, "Who are you?" I said, "Natasha." Mom just looked at me like I was crazy. I guess I shouldn't say that, but she doesn't know me. She thought at one time I was her sister. I told her, "No, I'm your daughter." She just looks at me blankly. I hate afternoons; Mother gets sundowner's bad. She doesn't remember Daddy at all. She thinks that Daddy died flying his plane and that it hit a tree. Where she got that, I have no idea. But Mother believes it. She's in her room probably putting on her gown. I told her we were going to have company. She put it on anyway. Oh well, it's better to let her do it than get upset. She is so demanding. Does not ask in a nice way, just tells you. I just say, "Yes, maham." She ate some supper and now is eating a banana. She will at least eat three or four bananas a day. It's so funny; she will eat not eat anything but the same cereal, etc.

Mother thinks she has a car; she never drove a car. She just told me she was going to sell it. I just look at her. Oh well, if she believes it, whatever. We watched the shows *Welk* and *Keeping Up* was one I have not seen. She went to bed. We had a tussle over the black pants. I have to sneak in after she goes to sleep, or she will get dressed in the middle of the night. She had her little money purse in the pocket of her pants. I told her to hide it, so I guess she did. She slept well. I hope it goes well for my sister today. As soon as she comes, I'm off like a prom dress.

05/23/10. We shall see what today brings. I've been up since 3:30 a.m. just thinking. My thoughts are killing me. I worry so much about my family. Mother does need to be somewhere like a nursing home. She needs good care 24-7. It's too hard for one person.

Mother asks me "Are you going to give me my bath?" when she gets up first thing. I told her, "No, Yvonne does that when she comes." Mother ate her breakfast—not so well for me. Mother kept saying, "When is Betty Crocker coming?" That's what she calls Yvonne. I told her she will be here soon. Yvonne came and gave her her bath. Mother was happy. Mother ate a good lunch and wanted to know when I was going home. Yvonne told her I was staying until tomorrow; she didn't say anything, just gave me the look. Mother stayed up until 10:00 p.m. watching TV. I slept in the bedroom, and Yvonne slept on the couch.

05/24/10. Yvonne woke me up at 5:45 a.m. and said that Doug, my brother, is coming. I'm so tired; I drank two cups of coffee. I feel like I have sand in my eyes. Mother slept until 8:45 a.m. We got ready and went to court. No other siblings showed up. Mother is going to the nursing home. I think she knows what is going on. We went down to the DMV to see whose name is on the trailer. Well, no trailer is in my mother's name or anyone's name. I know I gave them the title. I have no idea what happened. I'm so depressed over all this. I love her so much even though she doesn't know me. This is a hard decision. My sister tried so hard to keep her out of the nursing home even with Doug's and my help. Doug was so faithful in coming Monday and Tuesday; he was so kind and gentle with Mother. I could see the love in my brother's eyes that he has for her. This seems so unfair. I hate this disease. Why did this happen to such a kind and loving lady? My fibromyalgia is in a crisis today. I hurt all over. My muscles feel like I've been beaten.

Mother is quiet today. She asked me, "Is Betty Crocker [Yvonne] coming over?" I said yes and that I was staying also. I told her Doug was coming tomorrow, and I was going home.

06/11/10. Yvonne called me this morning. She said that the Mount Ida Nursing Home has an opening. She asks me if I wanted to come and go with her. I told her I would have to see how I felt. Too much driving.

06/08/10. Well when I got to Mother's, she didn't say much. She was watching TV, *The Price is Right*.

My sister and I went to the nursing home; my brother Doug was with Mother. The place was nice; loved the decor, very clean. It was very big, holds 120 residents. I only have one problem; one door does not have an alarm. They can't open the door on the southwest side. I hope that's true; I worry about her wandering out in the heat or cold. I know Mother doesn't want to go to the nursing home, but she drains us.

When we got back, she was asleep. She slept for a while.

Finally woke up for supper. Then Doug left, and all hell broke lose. Mother started saying over and over, "Who are you? Do you have children? Are you married? What is your husband's name?" I just lost it. I said, "Mother, yes, I have children, but you don't remember them. If I say Dale's first name, you remember his last name. Why can't you remember my name?" I hope the Lord will forgive me. I don't like to talk to my mother like that.

I had to take her teeth and hide them because she will lose them. She gets pretty upset with you when you take her choppers. Mother went to bed. Now wait about an hour and get her clothes, or she'll get dressed during the night. I hope she doesn't wake up during the night. I'm so tired, maybe because I drove three hours to get here. Good night, I hope, Momma.

06/09/10. I woke up at 2:30 a.m. Why? Who knows. My mind was racing, couldn't go back to sleep. I killed a bug, heard a lot of noises. Mother was up and down saying, "Where are my clothes in the washing machine? I'll put them in the dryer soon." At one time, Mother got her clothes; I had to get them away from her. I think we finally got up at 7:00 a.m. She ate breakfast. And now the twenty questions start; I told her no children, no husband. Mother looked at me for a while; I knew her mind was thinking hard. She asks me, "Do you have a friend?" I said, "No, I'm a lesbian." She looked at me, and we both started laughing. This place is like a zoo; you have Rackie the raccoon and his mother. Now that thing is on steroids; I'm scared of that thing. It gets very aggressive like "Open the door, bitch, let me in."

I went into the kitchen and saw a lizard on the floor. Thought I was going to have a heart attack; I just left it alone. One more animal will be okay, just feed and give him water. Does that sound normal to you? *We feed everything, all the li'l critters.* Makes the time fly.

You can't fix yourself anything to eat.

"Are you fixing my lunch?"

"No, Mama, I'm fixing my breakfast."

"Well, you know what I eat?"

"Yes, Mama."

06/10/10. She slept until five thirty this morning; she went to the bathroom. She asked me, "Is it time to get up?" I said, "No, not until eight a.m., Mama." She went back to sleep. I woke her up at 8:00 a.m. She was very aggressive with her breakfast being made. She is very demanding. I was so upset; she can be so trying on my nerves. Yvonne called me and said it would be noon before she would come. I was like "Okay, wanted to leave, had to stay." Mother said her usual "Who are you? Do you have a husband? Do you have any children?" I would answer no. I didn't want to go to "What are their names?" etc. She is so feeble, bent over more. I tried to have her stand up straight; she couldn't. Trying to put her sweater on was awful. It seems like she can't bend her arms. I think she needs physical therapy. Of course, she's ninety years old and stiff. Yvonne finally came over; I was so happy. I know she is tired and needed a break. I was so tired mentally and physically and have a three-hour drive ahead of me.

07/02/10. Got to Mother's at 1:00 p.m. She was watching TV, a Western. She was okay, not so confused. She did her usual "Who are you? Don't remember having you." I told her I was Daddy's. Mother, for some reason, thinks Daddy died when he flew his plane into a tree and he burned up. I just look at her like a deer in the headlights. She started wanting to go to bed at 5:00 p.m. I said, "No, I haven't given you your bedtime medicine yet." I reminded her to watch her *Wheel of Fortune*. She went to bed at 8:00 p.m. I took her teeth and sneaked in to take her clothes. She has a habit of spitting out the apple that she hasn't chewed up. That is so disgusting. I told her to spit it in the commode and flush it; she just looks at me. I hope she sleeps tonight. I'm tired from driving up from Crossett. Good night, I hope.

07/03/10. Mother slept well, got up only once last night. I had to remind her where her clothes were. She had put on another gown. She had underwear on the bed, which smelled of urine, but they were dry. Can't figure that one out unless she wet herself on the way to the bathroom. She didn't eat much cereal, ate the rest and a banana. She said the same things, "Who are you and where do you live?" "Is that your car outside?" etc. Well the sundowner's kicked in; she became demanding and kept saying "I'm going to bed."

"Not yet, Willie, you have to eat and watch your TV shows."

"Oh," she says.

I told her, "You haven't taken your medicine yet either."

Good one day, bad the next. She will be in the nursing home soon. I hope they are not mean to her. She will be out of there faster than a cat can lick his butt. Well, we watched her shows, and she went to bed

08/28/10. It was different; we took her to the dentist because of her bottom teeth hurting. Well, when we were coming in the dentist's office, she was going down and I couldn't hold her. A real nice man helped get her in the office. That was so awful liked to have killed me. My sister pulled the car closer to the door when we left.

Then we had to go to Walmart to pick up my meds. When my sister was getting the car, Mother was hanging on the pole outside the place. I said that never again would I do this.

I really haven't written anything about my mom; it's always the same. "Who are you, do you have any children?" But I have noticed she is feebler and she is bent over.

08/27/10. Mother has been falling a lot. My sister has been calling my brother to help get her up. Well, I told my sister that if she falls on me, I'm calling 911. Well sure enough, that afternoon after my sister left about three hours, Mother was coming out of the bathroom and I was in front of her. She kept going down, pulling me down with her. Well, on the floor we went; I broke her fall. I said, "Mother, I can't get you up, so I'm calling 911." They came, put her to bed, checked her vital signs; they were fine. They told Mother not to get out of bed. She said okay. She slept well, woke up a different woman. I can't figure her out.

08/29/10. Yvonne came over to stay, also because I was leaving to go to Springdale, then leaving to go to Mo. Mother didn't like me here, kept asking my sister when I was leaving. Then she really hurt my feelings when she said, "I like you" while pointing to my sister and just glaring at me. So I said, "Why do I come up?" she hates me for some strange reason.

Well, she was a little mean that day. But I was getting my stuff ready to leave in the morning.

08/30/10. Left to go to Springdale. Yeah.

09/05/10. My sister called me and said that she had to call Doug to come and pick Mother out of the floor and that she had bowel movement everywhere. My sister cleaned her up before my brother got there. He put her in bed.

09/06/10. My sister had to call my brother again at 4:00 a.m. She went to check on Mother, and she was on the floor and had had a bowel movement. She was in a mess. She had to call Doug to come and help get her up. She had already cleaned her up. Mother can't stay in her bedroom anymore. She gets up and falls.

09/07/10. I stopped by and saw Mother. My sister had an MD appointment for Mother. I hope she'll get in quick. I told my sister I would come up on September 8, 2010, and she is to call me and let me know what the MD said. Well, my sister called and said that the MD said Mother has two months to live.

09/08/10. We now have a hospital bed, and home health is to come and evaluate Mom. They are to get a catheter urine specimen. Mother does not like the pull-ups or the hospital bed.

We told her we can't pick her up or pull her anymore. She didn't understand, as usual. But on a funny note, my sister said that my brother Doug could just almost carry her well no. Mother fell going down the stairs; going to the car fell in the car was so muddy. My sister told the MD that we brought her mud and all; she just laughed and said that was okay. Then getting her back up the stairs was a hoot; my nephew had to come and get her up the stairs. I would have loved to see that.

09/09/10. My sister woke me up, and we changed Mother. The pull-up wasn't that wet.

She ate some oatmeal and took her meds. Doesn't seem to be as alert today. We changed her, and her pull-up was soaked, but her urine is dark. The home health nurse is coming today; I will write more lately. The home health nurse came; we talked and decided on hospice. They could give more care for Mother. The hospice nurse was very nice and explained everything to us. I think we will be more satisfied with the hospice. Mother had two bowel movements; it's been a long time since I cleaned someone up. It wasn't easy either. Boy, she was full of it. I hope she waits until I come back from Crossett this Sunday.

09/10/10. Mother was doing okay this morning. I'm leaving today, going home for the weekend. I'll leave Sunday. My husband is so good with me coming up here and staying like I do. He knows how much my mother means to me. As everyone, some will help, some won't. I hope eventually they will one wants money to come and with his own mother. I'm leaving to go back home. Will be back Friday. Two social workers came by and visited us. Mother slept well last night.

09/13/10. Came back to my mother's. The drive is always the same, boring. People were actually decent on the highway, which meant no road rage for me.

I saw how Mother was getting feebler. She can't walk. Now in Mother's head she still can she wants up all the time. That will drive you crazy. And you have to pull her up in the all the time. I just do it 'cause if you don't, she will drive you nuts.

09/14/10. Doug was here today and yesterday. He was really a great help to us pulling her up in the bed. Mother kept saying to my sister, who sleeps on the couch by Mother's bed, Mother told her to and sees what I have. That made Yvonne curious; somehow Mother had taken her diaper off. Yvonne said that the diaper was so heavy with urine; the nurse said that the diaper has gel in it that makes it feel heavy. We talked to the nurse and asked her different things. She is filling in for the regular nurse. We were really pleased with everything except the crazy bed. I hope we get a new one soon. I noticed how good she was sitting up for the hospice aide than for us. Maybe it was a better day for her. Yeah, probably so. She's pulling her diaper apart; I've been getting on her for that.

09/15/10. Mother is in a weird mood today. The aide came today and gave Mother her bath and changed the bed linens. They wash Mother's hair two times a week. She doesn't like getting her head washed.

The aide was really nice to Mother. She is very sweet woman. That really upsets me about Mother; she pulls at her diaper and pulls them apart. I tell her that that's not nice. So see, that's what you put up why when they can't walk anymore. The chaplain came by, and we talked and had a prayer before she left. So far I like them, but don't piss me off. My other sister came down and talked to Mother for a while. Doug was trying to fix the commode. Mother is going downhill fast. I hope she knows how much I love her. Mother's urine is so dark.

09/16/10. This is going to be a hell of a day. Mother has already started, didn't want to eat. Her usual that are you, "Are you married?" and "Do you have children?" I left and went to Walmart. Walking around the store was awesome.

Mother was still the same when I came back. I have learned to ignore her; now I must say that that is very hard.

09/17/10. Well, we woke up with a surprise. Mother threw her diaper on the floor with feces in it; boy, was that a wake-up call. So we had to watch her like a hawk. Every time she puts her hands in her lower area, we tell her, "Mother, what you are doing?"

"Nothing," she would say. Yeah, sure, Mother. My mother is a sneaky little woman.

09/18/10. This day was pretty good. Mother was the same, not throwing the diaper. Trying to get her to eat and drink is the problem. She will only eat three bites of food and maybe an ounce of water; that worries me so much. But I know the time will come. She is always pulling and trying to take that diaper off. Mother doesn't look like herself. I know she doesn't think like herself. She has no thinking process. She keeps us on our toes all the time.

09/19/10. I drove home today; I had to exchange vehicles with my husband. He needed my car for a trip this coming weekend. I hate leaving my sister, but my brother will help her if she needs it.

09/20/10. Well, I'm driving up to Mom's in the truck. I don't know if I dread it or know I should because she's my mom. I'm supposed to take care of her, that's the way it is supposed to be. I get so upset when Mother asks me to go to her bedroom. I try to explain to her the reason why, but her eyes are so sad, I want to cry. She can't understand, and I get so upset. I hate this disease; it has taken my mother away from me.

09/21/10. Another day with Mother; I wish she knew me. I have to tell her, and she has this blank look on her face. I think she tries sometimes to remember, but can't. She just looks at her shows. Does she really know what she is thinking? I think now she doesn't really know, or does she? She not eating that worries me, but my sister is so concerned. Yvonne would feed the world. I know her body is shutting down. My mother doesn't want to eat, doesn't have the appetite anymore. I know my mother will just waste away; I hope God will take her first. I hate watching her waste away, but she doesn't know it. I know that makes no sense. I try and we all do the right thing, but it is very hard to see her like this.

She's our child that we take care of now. We change her diapers; the aide gives her a bed to sleep in, but we have been alternating in turning her from side to side. You have to have two people now to do it; it is really hard on my back and my fingers for some reason.

The aide came to give her the daily bed bath since she can't get up now. Her aide is so good to her. Mother really likes her. After Yvonne left, my other sister came down for a visit. They will not be in the same room together. I just all of us put our differences aside for Mother's sake.

09/22/10. My sister fed my mother breakfast this morning. She only ate a few bites as usual and drank a few sips. Always wanting to go back to her room even though she is unable to walk, bless her heart. Mother is going down so fast. I hate this disease. Why did this happen to her? My brother is here to help with Mother. He has really been a good brother; he will hold Mother up while we change her. Not many men would do that, but he has stepped up and helps with his mother. Nothing unusual today.

09/23/10. Mother is getting weaker every day; it's so hard to see her this way. To see a sweet, hardworking, and caring woman get to barely being able to talk is so hard. We do what we can to make her comfortable. I don't think she is in pain. We ask and she says no; does she really mean it? I don't have a clue with this disease. Mother's voice is getting weaker; it breaks my heart to see her this way.

09/24/10. It's the same day; she is the same, eats some few bites, drinks sips of water, Carnation Breakfast Essentials, and eats some cream of wheat. We still turn her every two hours. She looks like she does not know what we are saying or understand what we are doing. We try so hard to understand this disease. It takes all the breath out of your lungs; your heart hurts, feels like it's breaking in two. Mother eats very little now. She doesn't talk very much at times. I look at her at times and wonder why this happened to her. She is such a sweet person. I have to go back home; Dale had to go out of town. I hated leaving my sister by herself, but I know if she needed help, my brother Doug will help her.

09/27/10. When I walked in Mother's today, I was shocked; her color was awful. I freaked out. She had the death look; I know that sounds crazy, but I've been a nurse for forty years. I had to settle myself down. My brother was upset; he had a rash on his back. Well it turns out he has shingles from stress. I traveled three hours today, and I guess I was tired. We are stressed out. My brother Doug is so good with Mother. He is so gentle with her; not many sons would be that way. Mother still doesn't eat or drink much anymore. She gets strangled when she drinks. Only the water, not the Carnation Breakfast Essentials. We give her medication one pill at a time.

09/28/10. I found out that the worse thing is when you have to get into nurse mode with your mother. I had to give my mother an enema and dig out an impaction. That is for someone else to do; that's your mother. I do it because I love her and she needed help. She took care of me and my siblings. I know if she was in her right mind, it would have upset her to think I had to do that to her. She was a private woman, didn't want her children in trouble that Mother would hide things from Daddy. This disease takes everything good that my mother would never do that. Until this disease is cured, others will have to go through what my family is going through.

09/29/10. I woke up at 6:00 a.m. I saw a light on in the living room; Yvonne was making coffee. Mother was sleeping. I have to drink my coffee in the morning. I drank my coffee, turned on the TV. Looking at Mother, she didn't say a word. I just watched her, wondering if she is sleeping. I hope they are dreams she can understand, back when she was a child or something. Good things. I think what is so heartbreaking is, she does not know her grandchildren. Jackie said, "Mother, I have my memories in my head of Grandma. She raised me, I lived with them until Paw had his stroke." My daddy said that I worked from 7:00 a.m. to 3:00 p.m. at the hospital in Hot Springs, and Jackie had colic. I was up most of the night due to her crying. My daddy was so worried about my health; he told me to get her on my days off, and they would keep her when I worked. She said, "Nothing can take them away from me."

Jackie came to see Mother; she lives in Missouri. Jackie told me, "I want you to know that hospice nurses and social workers will routinely have meetings about Grandma. The doctors are not out in the homes with the clients. You want to make changes, and you don't know how this is going to affect the families that we see day in and day out. We have the report with the families, not you." Jackie is a social worker; she has a master's degree. She entered a hospice in Northwest Arkansas.

09/30/10. I'm awake at 4:00 a.m. I don't know why. I went into the living room, checked on Mother and my sister. I even called my husband and woke him up, don't know why. I started writing down things about Mother. My computer was in the living room, and I didn't want to wake them up. I heard something outside growling. I turned off the light; it scared me. I accidentally woke my sister up at 5:00 a.m. trying to get my cell phone charger. I went back to my room. She came in and said, "Why are you up so early?" I said that I felt something wasn't right and I heard something growling outside. I was writing in my journal also. Before Yvonne was going to feed Mother, we checked her to change her diaper. I pulled the covers back; the smell was awful. I put Vicks salve up my nose; she had the worse bowel movement I have ever seen in my life. I could smell blood in her bowel movement; it was everywhere. I was freaking out. I do this dance that I don't want to do this and I hate the smell of blood in feces. It's a horrible smell. Mother was listless, would not respond, refused to eat, did not even open her eyes to look at her shows. Mother responded by saying "Uh-huh" or "No"; that went on until noon. I asked her, "Willie, do you want some milk shake?" She said, "Yes." I ran to the fridge and got her one. She drank several sips. She ate six bites for lunch; that is encouraging. The nurse came to check Mother. We pointed out that her big toes are red; she ordered fungal powder. The grandchildren came to visit—Jackie, Raye, and Daniel. It really affected Jackie today; she went outside and cried. I went out, and she kept saying, "I'm sorry, Mom." I told her, "It's okay." I was crying also it's okay. Jackie lost her other grandmother one year ago in April. Raye and Daniel also lost their other grandmother not even a year ago. It's so hard on them seeing Grandma like this and knowing what's going to happen soon. For supper Mother ate only four bites. This is so trying on all of us. Can't eat or sleep. We have to keep our health up to take care of Mother. Mother looking at the TV her head of her bed is up. Now her eyes are closed. I told Evelyn, my other sister, when I called her about Mother today. I told her we will act like a family for Mother's sake. We may not like each other, but we will for Mother. It's so stupid how things happen, but we will put our feelings aside for Mother. My sister agreed. I told her if Yvonne is here and she wants to visit, Yvonne will walk out and I'll be in here with her. Lord, why do these things happen? Families are so whacked. We turn Mother every two hours, always. It's getting to my neck and back, though, but anything for my mother. Mother did a lot for us when we were children. So suck it up for Mom.

10/01/10. Sister woke me up at 6:45 a.m. She made me coffee; she always does that. Sister says she's glad I'm here. Before my sister feeds Mother, we check her, and another big surprise bowel movement. Mother ate five bites of oatmeal this morning. I ask her, "Do you love me, Mother?" instead of calling her Willie. She said yes—well, she shook her head up and down. Surely she wasn't head banging. We listen to country music. Cindy, Mother's aide, brought her some flowers today. They are so pretty. We found her a vase and put them in front of the TV so she can see them. At lunch, she didn't want to eat, only sleep. I told my sister to go at 1:00 p.m. and do what she had to do at her house.

My other sister came down when she saw that sister was gone. She asks Mother, "Do you know who I am?" Mother said, "Jennifer." My other sister said, "No, I'm Jennifer's mother," and she said her name. I gave Mother some milk shake; she drank a lot. Then Yvonne drove up. My other sister left; they don't speak. It breaks my heart. We have to take our pride or whatever, put it aside for Mother's sake; she agreed. Mother didn't eat much of her oatmeal for supper. We turned her. It's hard; we change her a lot. The bowel movements are loose and smell horrible. We place pillows between her legs and behind her back. Good night, Mother.

10/02/10. Sister had coffee ready this morning. Sister checked Mother. She had this weird bowel movement; it was small. And Mother had urinated also. She only ate four bites of oatmeal for breakfast. We turned her and turned on CMT. Mother talked more and wants to go into her bedroom. I wish we could.

Vicks salve works wonders on me when we change Mother. Mother had a bowel movement around noon. Sister left around noon after we cleaned Mother up. Sometimes we get crap everywhere. We just laugh and go on and do what we have to do. Sister left, and the other sister came down. Mother wasn't as responsive to her. We sat and talked; I told her that my sister wanted me to do Mother's obit. She said sister isn't going to get all she wants because when Mother is gone, so is her guardianship. I just said I'm just trying to be the peacemaker. I did ask her questions, for which she gave me the answers. Sister came back; the other sister left. Mother ate two bites for lunch. I took a nap. When I woke up, I told sister I thought I would go to Walmart. Sister said, "Let's turn and check Mother." I said, "Okay." I was eating candy corn when she loosened Mother's diaper; I almost choked. I said, "Thanks, sister, I will never them again." Mother had a horrible bowel movement. We cleaned her up. My sister and I laugh or cry about things. I enjoyed my trip to Walmart, believe it or not, crazy people and all. Got back to Mother's, and sister said she only ate three bites of oatmeal. We give her water all the time, but she will only drink a few swallows. We checked Mother before we turned her; she wasn't wet, but we cleaned her who hah (that's what Mother and I would call her vagina). It was a joke between me and her.

Mother asked for her glasses; I was so surprised. I love it! I asked her if she wanted to watch *Keeping Up*. She said yes. Don't think she did though. She's sleeping now. We will change her before we go to bed. Then tomorrow we start all over again.

Good night, Mother.

10/03/10. Sister woke me up at 6:30 a.m., said Mother had a bowel movement. I ask her, "Please let me have a cup of coffee before we get started." We could hear something crying like an animal of sorts. Could not figure out where it was coming from. We cleaned Mother up. She only ate one bite of oatmeal and would not drink anything. She did drink water with meds but would not drink any extra. Mother's rectum was red, so we put aloe vera on it. We turned her again. Today we cleaned; it was fun—*not!* Something to keep busy. Mother would answer me when I would say something to her.

I don't think my brother should come; he has shingles. So I cancelled my appointment for Tuesday. He will have to come Wednesday. I have an appointment with a shrink in Monticello for my disability. Sister is going to feed Mother now for lunch. Mother said yes. I hope she eats something. One bite down, some water, two bites, some water. Mother asks for some milk shake and drank several sips. I know the time is coming. I don't want it to everyone is different. I wish now she was up wandering around, asking me questions, and telling me things I really didn't want to know. I wish she was up wandering in her room. Mother is sleeping now. I hope she wakes up at 2:00 p.m. and does her sundowner's thing.

Well, other sister and her grandsons came down. Mother said a few words to her, then went back to sleep. I ask other sister about a preacher to preach in Mother's funeral. She gave me a suggestion. I ask her about pictures that she should be in. This is so weird for me. When the great-granddaughter came, Mother roused. She had helped take care of Mother. When I couldn't come, I would pay the great-granddaughter. If family can be friends and love each other through all this disease, it would be so much better. It's hard anyway so hard anyway, but when you don't get along, it's so nerve-racking. Mother has drank a few sips of milk shake. She keeps saying she wants to go into her room. I wish she could, bless her heart. I think back when I was a child; Mother would rub Vicks on my chest for a cold. Now I put the Vicks up my nose 'cause of my mother's bowel movements. That is so sad. She stares at the TV, but I don't know if she is really watching it or not. I'm really tired today, for some reason. Mother had another bowel movement. We cleaned her up, then went to bed.

Good night, Mother.

10/04/10. We woke up again, and it's the same every morning. Mother always has a weird bowel movement; Vicks again up the nose. That saved my life. Mother didn't eat. She had only one bite for breakfast. Mother has dark circles under her eyes. She has lost so much weight. Mother lies there with her eyes open; she just stares. We had a new aide come today. She was nice but not as good as Cindy. Mother had a wet diaper; we changed her. We change her position every two hours. I can't say that enough: her skin was good, no bed sores. She refused lunch, only drank one sip of water. Mother almost started crying. Seems every day is awful. Only a few of the grandchildren come to see Mother. What else is new? Mother wouldn't eat. She didn't say she wanted to go to her room or she wanted her clothes on, bless her heart. It just kills us that she can't now. We try so hard for us that she won't eat or drink. We take her blood pressure every day, sometimes twice. She drinks water, not so much with the eating. She keeps pulling her gown up; we pull it down. I keep saying, "Mother, what in the world are you doing?" She says, "I don't know."

We finally went to bed. Good night, Mother.

10/05/10. We are up early as usual to check on Mother and change her diaper. She doesn't talk much anymore; we turn her every two hours. Mother only eats a few bites. The hospice nurse and aide are so nice. Cindy is the aide, and Sandra is the nurse. We don't know what we would do without them. We raise Mother up in the bed well the head of the bed for her to watch TV. I don't know if she watches them or not.

Mother has her eyes closed most of the time. She'll smile every once in a while. What she's smiling at, I have no idea. She didn't eat much of the cream of wheat for supper. We changed Mother and got her ready for bed. Good night, Mother.

10/06/10. I have to go home. I have to see a physiologist for getting my disability. I don't want to leave. I'm afraid something will happen while I'm gone. My brother Doug will be with my sister while I'm gone.

10/08/10. I'm back. I missed not being here. I missed not being at home. I'm torn, but I have a good husband who understands. Mother is so bad. She doesn't talk much now. We give my mother good oral hygiene, can't stand a cruddy mouth. She looks blankly; I know that doesn't make much since, but it kills me. She doesn't want to eat or drink. We have to beg her to eat just a bite of oatmeal or cream of wheat. How we wish she was up and about, talking. Sister and I were up to 12:00 a.m. to 1:00 a.m. We talked about things. Mother doesn't respond anymore like she used to. At times she will. It's like a spark hits her brain, and she'll talk. Good night, Mother.

10/09/10. Mother started on Carnation drink today; she will not eat now. She drinks about half of it. I wish she would eat and drink more; I can't force it on her though. I have to look at her to make sure she's breathing. Her color is not good. Her blood pressure is low. She opens her eyes sometimes when I say "Willie." She gets to shaking sometimes. I go and put her hand on hers, and she stops shaking. She'll pull her gown up, and I'll pull it down. We would tell her, "No, Mother, don't do that." That goes on all day. The great-granddaughter came with the preacher to meet Mother. His wife is my late uncle's niece. Mother was more alert with this visit. We want him to preach on her funeral. Being that he's married to my uncle's niece, he's family.

Good night, Mother.

10/10/10. Today I was surprised. My husband came and visited me and Mother. I was so happy. He knew I needed him. Sometimes I think he doesn't care about my situation with my mother. We talked; he does know how I feel about my mother. I will stay here with my sister and my mother until the end. He understands and will be here for me. I'm so glad I have him. We went to Walmart and walked around and talked. Came back to Mother's sister, and I changed and turned Mother. Dale left and went back home. I really enjoyed his visit.

Good night, Mother.

10/11/10. Had to get up early. Brother comes today. He takes the garbage can down to the road. Cindy came and gave Mother a bath. Mother ate cream of wheat. Before her bath, Mother ate four or five bites of cream of wheat. Mother will drink some water with a lot of begging. Mother loves her milk shakes. Mother seems to respond better to brother. That's her baby boy, and she loves her baby boy, and he is so good with her. You can see the caring in his voice and the way he handles her; he loves his mother. I don't know if Mother will see her ninetieth birthday. I wish she could, but all the signs show that her body is shutting down.

Good night, Mother.

10/12/10. I'm just sitting, looking at my mother, who has these blank eyes. I don't know how much she knows or if she comprehends. I wish I could get into her mind for one day, see what she sees and hears and understands. My mother doesn't deserve these later years of her life. She would worry so much about everyone and everything. She didn't want anyone to be mad at anyone. I know that when Mother is in heaven, she will be normal again. No worries, just smiling all the time. She deserves that. Of anyone I know, my mother will have many crowns. I love her so much. I know I'm selfish, but I need to let her go to be with her loved ones in heaven. I hate funerals and all the processes of things that go with it. I know people want to be nice and show you how much they love you, but at the time, you want to be alone, or I do. I have guilt for over six year's time to let it go.

Good night, Mother.

10/13/10. I saw the light on in the kitchen. I got up, went to the bathroom. When I saw Mother, I went over to put my hand over her chest to make sure she was breathing. My sister came over. I told her I was I had to come over she was I told her I had to come over to over to see if she was alive. Sister said "I made her cream of wheat." It hit us as funny. We started laughing. It was like Mother was alive because sister made her cream of wheat. Lord, I think we are crazy. Mother ate a few bites this morning. Same routine. Cindy came this morning. Cindy gave her a bath. We turned Mother, turned on *The Price is Right* and *Jeopardy!* for Mother. Does she watch? I have no idea. I know she can hear them. Then *Spin the Wheel* comes on. I don't watch that show anymore. Sister is worried about Mother not eating so much. I think sister would die if she thought Mother was starving to death. It was the usual today.

Good night, Mother.

10/14/10. I'm sitting up in bed, writing this is on the sixteenth of October. I have no time to write. It's about 5:00 a.m. I can't sleep, so I write Mother's story. Mother wrote a book about growing up changed her sibling's names. I can't figure that out. Yet. Nothing new. The funniest thing is trying to get Mother's teeth out. Sister will explain to Mother to make the *whew* sound so air will get under her palate to release. Sister would make the sound, and Mother would repeat in her frail little voice. We would laugh to keep from crying. Mother didn't understand. I told my sister that if we get them damn teeth out, we were not putting them back in.

Good night, Mother.

10/15/10. This morning, Mother wasn't responsive. When Cindy gave her a bath, she still didn't respond. All throughout the bath, Mother didn't make a sound or say anything. Mother had a deep cough. I checked her lungs. I couldn't hear any fluid and could hear good breath sounds. Mother was coughing, so I told my sister to call the hospice nurse to come and check on her. The nurse came and checked Mother. We put booties on her heels. She keeps somehow getting them off.

She is like hoodie. Her voice is so frail. We put some thickener for her so she would not choke. The hospice nurse discontinued some of her meds. Mother has lost so much weight. She won't eat but will drink milk shakes. Mother sleeps all the time. Sometimes she will watch TV no much. Mother has drunk her milk shakes; her urine smells so bad. I don't know if it's because of her renal failure. It smells like she's had a bowel movement. I wonder if she's hurting or feels uncomfortable. I worry about her so much. We checked her diaper to see if she needed changing. Well, she had a massive bowel movement. If she doesn't bowel movement for a week she will be fine.

Good night, Mother.

10/16/10. It's 5:00 a.m. I'm awake, can't sleep, so I'm writing. I'm going to take a shower and get ready for the great day with Willie. Lord, have mercy. Did Mother have a surprise for us this morning? I've never in my life seen so much poop. I put Vicks up the nose and did my "Don't want to do" dance. So crazy, but that's how I do it. If Mother had her mind, she would call me crazy. I would, and I know my other sister and brother would. Mother, in her frail voice, said she wanted something to drink. It breaks my heart that she can't get up and go to her room. Mother all of a sudden said she had plenty of time. Then she said something was wrong with her panties. Mother said in a frail voice, "We have plenty of time." Sometimes she doesn't make sense. I don't think it will be long. She shakes her hands. We put our hands on hers and tell her it's going to be okay.

Heather came to visit Mother. She is the chosen one. Mother loves her the most. Heather was watching the Razorbacks game and giving Mother the play-by-play of the game. She had pulled a chair beside Mother's bed. I know Mother didn't understand a word, but Heather enjoyed being there. Heather left.

Sometimes Mother is awake. Most of the time, she does the strangest things like putting the sheet over her head. I pull it down.

Good night, Mother.

10/17/10. Sister got me up at 8:00 a.m. I drank a cup of coffee. We changed Mother; she had a great urine diaper. She drank her Carnation Breakfast Essentials. I gave her some lorazepam drops. We crushed her pills, took her blood pressure. She still has that blank look this morning. She slept most of the morning and was more awake all of a sudden. Heather came by to visit before she left to go back home. The other sister came down to visit while Heather was here. The other sister left before my sister came back. Mother talked well; she answered questions in her frail little voice. She complained of pain. I gave her lorazepam routinely. Mother looked at me with her pitiful eyes that I hate so bad. She got hot, and I took off her flannel gown. Heather left. She was crying. It hurts the girls so much; it will be over soon. Mother raised them. Raye Marie came by to visit also. I think it was good for Mother to have her grandchildren visit. Mother drank milk shake. She was saying something and holding her head. I bent down, a said her head hurt. Her blood pressure was 152/127. We gave her blood pressure meds, and I gave her the lorazepam. I checked her blood pressure thirty-five minutes later, and it was 120/67. I will check her pressure at different intervals. Mother is sleeping now. I gave her lorazepam because she was restless. Though it put her to sleep, she coughed some.

Good night, Mother.

10/18/10. Not a good morning. I don't know if Mother will make it through the day. She's not responsive. I ask her if she wants her bath, and she said no. I don't know what to do. I had a meltdown when my sister and I were changing and Mother had no response. I couldn't help it. I told my sister, "Wait, give me a minute. Then I'll be okay." I think this is the end of my diary. The hospice aide, Cindy, gave Mother her bath—no response. She is so fragile. Her temperature is 98ax.

I'm thinking I don't want to let go. But then you would think am I being selfish. Does she want to go? It's so hard to think about it. Am I a selfish person? I don't want her to go, but that's not my decision. I don't want her to suffer. I pray she isn't. I'm sitting here watching her breathe, watching her every move. She moves her arms and legs. "Maybe she will rally back now," I say, but she won't. I have this thing; I can tell.

Mother was restless. I asked her if she was hurting. She said yes. Her blood pressure was 112/66, pulse 90. I gave her lorazepam for pain. Again Mother was restless; we checked her. She had a bowel movement. We cleaned her up, but there was no response except one thing: "I want to wear," and that's all she said. I checked her lungs; they sounded wet. That may sound crazy, but that's the only way to explain it. The nurse came and checked Mother; her pulse oximeter read 95 percent, pulse 86, no temperature. Her respiratory rate was 38. She feels like it can be anytime when Mother will start to mottle her extremities. This is because the blood is going to the vital organs. Then the vital organs will shut down. The suction machine. The DME Company brought out a new one, but it was my fault. He fixed it for us. It's going to be a long night.

I called the other sister to come down; Mother's legs were getting mottled. All of us girls were there when Mother died at 11:55 p.m. I already miss her so much. I cried when I couldn't hear her heart beating. I heard her heart stop beating. I hugged and kissed her forehead.

Good-bye, Mother.

That was such a blessing for me to be able to hear her sweet little heart stop. I had a stethoscope. I bought several years ago.

I want all you families to please stand together. If your parents have Alzheimer's or dementia, stand together, don't fall apart. Make sure your parents have a will.

This is what happened to us. Our parents did not. I had to probate Mother's and Daddy's.

I have one sister and brother on my side. I also have a brother and sister who are not. I'm administrator over Mother's and Daddy's estate.

01/25/11. Today it seemed like a final act. My sister and I transferred Mother's account to the estate to me at the bank. Then I went to the real estate office and put the land up for sale.

Mother has nine acres, and Daddy has ten acres. I guess it's closure or the beginning of the fight. Since I probated Mother's and Daddy's land, I got a letter from my other sister's attorney. The letter said how the siblings should get together and discuss about the land and how Daddy wanted it in the family. I'm not so sure about that; he wouldn't want the hatred. It reminds me of Mother when she had her right mind. She told me that Granddaddy said he raised some greedy children. I think about that all the time. I feel like that's what my other brother and sister think about me. I really don't care; by law, the land had to be probated. My sister and I went to Mother's grave to see if the headstone had come or not. It was strange seeing her grave and her picture, and someone had put flowers on her grave. I have put things to rest. I wish we could get along no way. Just making the funeral arrangements was terrible. I don't know why the other sister and brother and their families hate my sister and me. I don't have to deal with them; I live in another city. I will move back to Hot Springs, and I will check on Mother's trailer. I will not put up with any mess from them, and neither will my husband.

It had been a long six years plus that the family had to take care of Mother. I miss her and Daddy so much, but they would want us to get along. I think Daddy knew what would happen. I wish he had left a will; since he didn't, I took the responsibility for having the crap hit the fan. Now you have to understand, I have some crazy people in my family.

Let me explain. I put the nineteen acres up for sale. I feel like that's the only fair way to settle things. If you try to split up the land, you know everyone will want the highway footage. That's for sure, I know.

My other sister didn't see my mother for nine months. She drove right past my mother's trailer in leaving and coming back to her own house. One time Mother asked me if my sister was still living up the hill. I told her yes. Mother asked me to call her; she wanted to see her. I did what Mother wanted. I called her and told her to come and see her mother; she was asking for her. I told her anytime I'm there she can see Mother because she will not come around my oldest sister. I found some old things about Mother that I wrote down, so I know it's confusing,

My mother was a peacemaker, didn't want any trouble. I can remember when Grandma Smith died. The family was giving her things that the other family had given her. I told Mother I wanted Grandma's sewing machine because Daddy and Mother had bought it for her. Mother told me that she thought Emma and Paul had bought it for Grandma. I told her, "No, it was you and Daddy." Well, she wouldn't ask anyone. Well, needless to say, the sewing machine was Mother's, and she gave it to my sister. Well, I have the sewing machine.

When Grandma was sick, the girls would take turns staying with her in her home until she died. I thought that was so loving of them. They loved Grandma, their mother.

I think back that is what if you can take care of your parents, but don't let it break you down. One person can't do it on your own. It was three of us for a long time. And it was for a year or more that my sister stayed day and night. I would come and relieve her on weekends, and Doug would relieve her on Mondays and Tuesdays. I really don't know how my sister has kept a sane mind. I know I personally couldn't. I would get so nervous when I would stay with Mother. I would say when I was driving up to stay, "You're not going to get upset with your mother, understand?" Well that never worked on me, I hate to say. It's been a train wreck, family members against each other.

I will not ever forget when we were making the arrangements for Mother. The one brother wouldn't even come into the room. He sent his daughter and granddaughter in to listen and report back to him, and he would say whether he liked it or not. Now I'm a very straightforward person. He didn't spend a dime on Mother's funeral. I really don't think he should have a say in anything. But he is Mother's son, so we grinned and bore it. I was all Xanaxed up for the occasion so my family wouldn't be so upset with my mouth.

I think I'm the most outspoken of the bunch. I listened to what the brother had his mouthpiece had to say, and we would talk about it. I was not surprised when the brother asked about Mother's ring that she gave to me. I told my niece that Mother would be buried with the ring. That seemed to calm them down. The other thing was Josh Turner's "Long Black Train" to be played at the funeral when they show the pictures at the funeral. I honestly didn't care. Mother loved that song and video. I knew the one song that was to be played was "Jesus Take Me Home." And it turned out well, thank goodness. I was well pleased with everything in general. Still the family was divided, not down the middle, but still divided.

I'm thinking that one of these days, maybe we will be a complete family. The Fourth of July was a special time for us when we were growing up. We wanted it to be that way again.

Life goes on for the living. Visit the grave often, tell them how much you love and miss them. I bought three plots: one for Mother and one for me and one for my husband. I'm in the middle, so I'll have the ones I love close by.

Try not to be enemies with your family.

That's my mother's story with the disease that took her away from her family. All of Mother's memories of her children and grandchildren. It really helps if you write down every day what you have with your family member. Keep a diary like me. It does help when you read over what happened and how the disease has progressed. How your family member reacts to you. They will either know you or ask who you are. I found that with Mother, she knew some family but couldn't remember their names. Like me, Mother couldn't remember my name.

The End